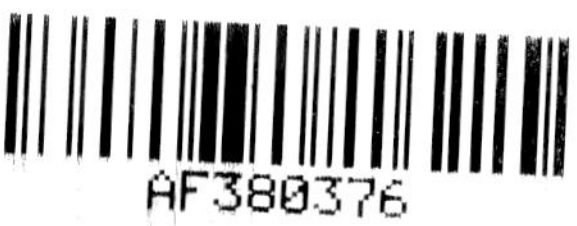

This Notebook Belongs To:

____

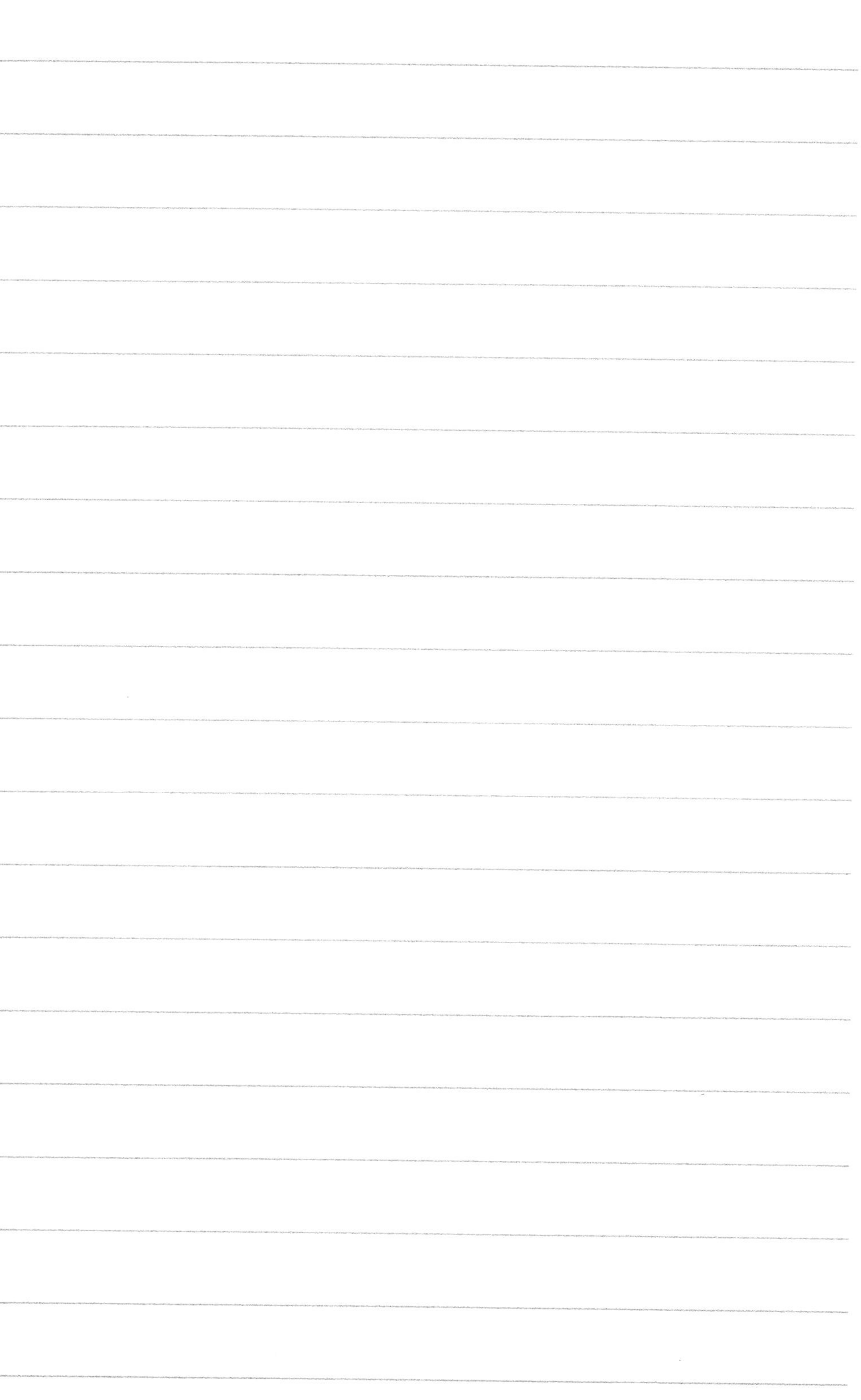

Made in the USA
Monee, IL
07 July 2026

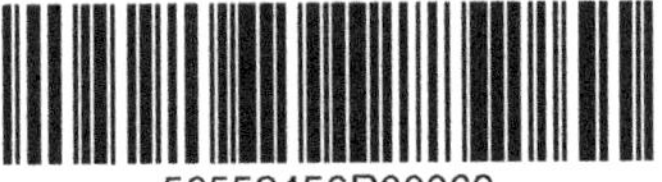

56552456R00069